MIND DIET

FOOD LIST

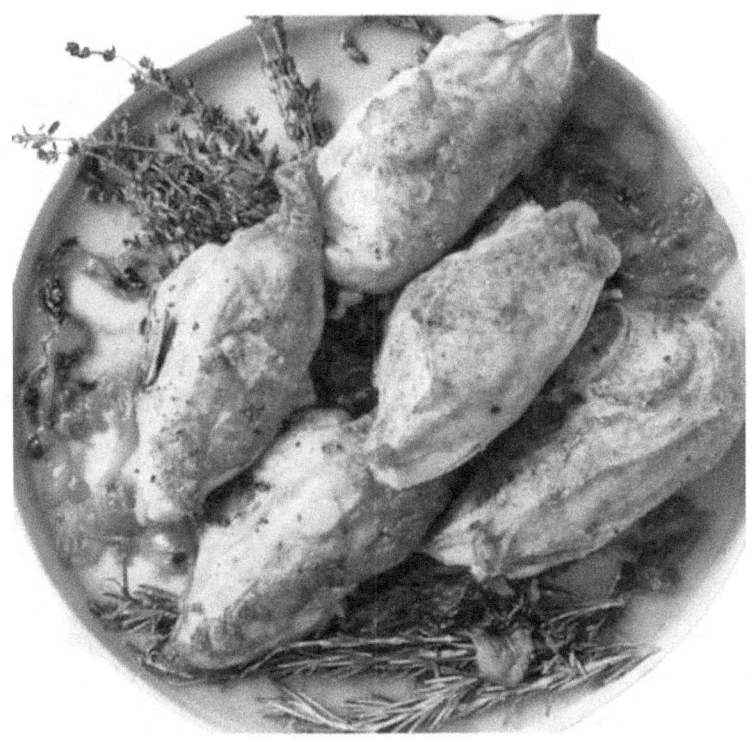

LYSANDRA QUINN

Contact the Author

Thank you for reading my book! I would love to hear from you, whether you have feedback, questions, or just want to share your thoughts. Your feedback means a lot to me and helps me improve as a writer.

Please don't hesitate to reach out to me through

contactmelysandraquinn@gmail.com

I look forward to connecting with my readers and appreciate your support in this literary journey. Your thoughts and comments are valuable to me.

OTHER BOOKS BY THE AUTHOR

SLOW COOKER MIND DIET COOKBOOK

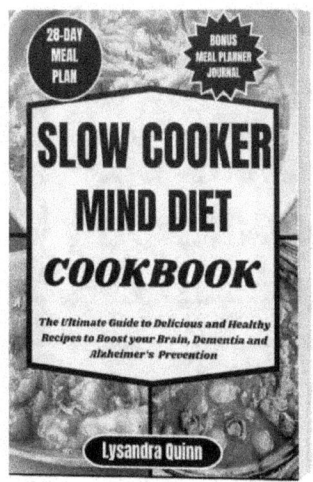

MIND DIET NINJA AIRFRYER COOKBOOK

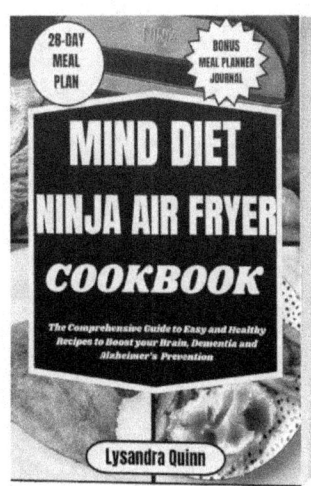

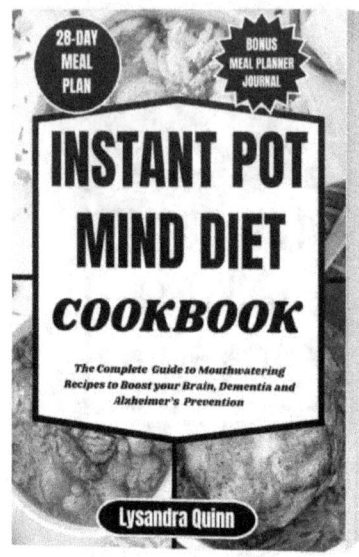

TABLE OF CONTENTS

INTRODUCTION

In the quiet corners of our lives, where whispers of health concerns linger, there exists a profound yearning for solutions that transcend the ordinary. This is a tale of discovery, a narrative woven with the delicate threads of hope and resilience, where the MIND diet emerges as a beacon of light in the shadowy realm of cognitive well-being.

Picture this: a bustling kitchen, the air saturated with the aromatic dance of herbs and spices. Pots clink, knives tap, and the symphony of culinary creation unfolds. Amidst this culinary cacophony, there lies a profound revelation – the transformative power of the MIND diet. The story begins not with sterile statistics or clinical jargon but with the beating hearts of individuals whose lives have been touched by the alchemy of carefully curated ingredients.

In the vast tapestry of dietary regimens, many have wandered, seeking solace for minds besieged by the specter of cognitive decline. Countless have traversed the labyrinth of nutrition, their hopes flickering like fragile flames in the face of an impending storm. The struggle is real, and so is the desperation that accompanies the quest for a remedy. Yet, in this labyrinth of uncertainty, the MIND diet emerges as a steadfast guide, a compass pointing towards cognitive vitality.

As a seasoned dietician with a tapestry of experiences spanning decades, I found myself drawn into the enigmatic world of the MIND diet. The dangers lurking in the shadows of cognitive decline were too palpable to ignore, and the need for a beacon of hope became imperative. Thus began my odyssey – a relentless pursuit of knowledge, an exploration of the culinary landscape that held the promise of preserving the sanctity of the mind.

The danger of neglecting cognitive health is akin to navigating treacherous waters without a compass. Alzheimer's disease and related neurodegenerative conditions cast long shadows over the lives of millions, stealing not just memories but the very essence of identity. The urgency to unravel the mysteries of these afflictions became my driving force, propelling me into the realms of scientific research and nutritional expertise.

The MIND diet, an acronym for the Mediterranean-DASH Diet Intervention for Neurodegenerative Delay, emerged as a revelation in my journey. Beyond the confines of a clinical term, it became a lifeline for those teetering on the precipice of cognitive decline. The fusion of the Mediterranean and DASH diets birthed a culinary masterpiece designed not just for sustenance but as a shield against the ravages of time on the mind.

But how did this culinary concoction transform the lives of those who embraced it? Picture faces illuminated by the glow of regained clarity, the twinkle returning to eyes once clouded by uncertainty. As a dietician, witnessing this metamorphosis was nothing short of witnessing a miracle.

"Why had we not stumbled upon this sooner?" This question echoes through the corridors of time, resonating with the collective lament of those who, in their pursuit of health, traversed landscapes barren of answers. The MIND diet, with its repertoire of brain-boosting foods – berries, leafy greens, nuts, and fish – stands as a testament to the resilience of the human spirit and the power of informed nutrition.

But this is not just a tale of dangers averted; it is a symphony of benefits, a crescendo of advantages that echo through the lives touched by the MIND diet. Improved cognitive function, heightened memory retention, and a shield against the encroaching fog of forgetfulness – these are the notes composing the melody of rejuvenated minds.

As I delved deeper into the annals of nutritional science, the advantages of the MIND diet became increasingly apparent. Beyond the immediate benefits of cognitive preservation, this culinary symphony orchestrated a myriad of positive outcomes – cardiovascular health, weight management, and the fortification of the immune system. The ripple effect of mindful eating extends far beyond the boundaries of the mind, resonating through the entirety of one's well-being.

Consider this not merely as a collection of recipes but as a narrative, a dialogue with your body and mind. The MIND diet is not a mere list of ingredients but a love letter to your well-being, each dish crafted with the precision of a poet, the care of an artist, and the wisdom of a seasoned dietician.

As you embark on this culinary journey, ask yourself: What is the true cost of neglecting the well-being of your mind? Can you put a price on the richness of your memories, the clarity of your thoughts, and the vitality of your spirit? The MIND diet is not just a guide; it is an invitation to reclaim the narrative of your cognitive health, to pen a story of resilience and triumph.

In the pages that follow, you will not find mere recipes; you will discover a roadmap to cognitive vitality. Each ingredient is a brushstroke, each dish a canvas upon which you paint the portrait of your well-being. Join me in this odyssey, where the alchemy of nutrition meets the poetry of culinary creation and let the MIND diet be the pen that inscribes the chapters of a healthier, more vibrant life.

CHAPTER 1

WHAT IS THE MIND DIET?

The Mind Diet, short for the MIND diet (Mediterranean-DASH Diet Intervention for Neurodegenerative Delay), is a dietary approach designed to promote brain health and reduce the risk of cognitive decline. Developed by researchers, this eating plan combines elements of the Mediterranean and DASH (Dietary Approaches to Stop Hypertension) diets. The Mind Diet emphasizes foods that are rich in nutrients beneficial for brain function and has gained attention for its potential to support cognitive well-being.

Importance of Nutrition for Brain Health

Nutrition plays a crucial role in maintaining optimal brain health. The brain requires a variety of nutrients, including vitamins, minerals, antioxidants, and omega-3 fatty acids, to function properly. A well-balanced and nutrient-dense diet can support cognitive function, enhance memory, and reduce the risk of neurodegenerative diseases. Understanding the importance of nutrition for brain health underscores the significance of making mindful and nutritious food choices.

Principles of the Mind Diet

The Mind Diet is based on several key principles that prioritize specific food groups associated with cognitive benefits. These principles include a focus on berries, leafy greens, nuts, whole grains, fish, and poultry, while limiting the intake of red meat, butter, cheese, and sweets. The diet encourages a holistic approach to nutrition, combining elements from proven dietary strategies to create a comprehensive plan aimed at nourishing the brain.

Key Components of a Mind-Healthy Diet

A mind-healthy diet is characterized by the inclusion of nutrient-rich foods that support cognitive function. Key components of the Mind Diet include:

- ✓ Fruits and Vegetables: Rich in antioxidants and vitamins.
- ✓ Whole Grains: Provide sustained energy and essential nutrients.
- ✓ Nuts: Source of healthy fats and antioxidants.
- ✓ Fish: High in omega-3 fatty acids, beneficial for brain health.
- ✓ Poultry: Lean protein for overall well-being.
- ✓ Olive Oil: Healthy monounsaturated fats with potential cognitive benefits.

CHAPTER 2

FRUITS

Blueberries:

Nutritional Information (per 1 cup):

- ✓ Calories: 84
- ✓ Fiber: 3.6g
- ✓ Vitamin C: 14mg
- ✓ Antioxidants: Anthocyanins

Strawberries:

Nutritional Information (per 1 cup, sliced):

- ✓ Calories: 53
- ✓ Fiber: 3g
- ✓ Vitamin C: 89mg
- ✓ Antioxidants: Ellagic acid

Blackberries:

Nutritional Information (per 1 cup):

- ✓ Calories: 62
- ✓ Fiber: 7.6g
- ✓ Vitamin C: 30mg
- ✓ Antioxidants: Anthocyanins

Raspberries:

Nutritional Information (per 1 cup):

- ✓ Calories: 64
- ✓ Fiber: 8g
- ✓ Vitamin C: 32mg
- ✓ Antioxidants: Quercetin

Oranges:

Nutritional Information (per medium orange):

- ✓ Calories: 62
- ✓ Fiber: 3.1g
- ✓ Vitamin C: 70mg
- ✓ Antioxidants: Citrus flavonoids

Grapes:

Nutritional Information (per 1 cup, red or green):

- ✓ Calories: 104
- ✓ Fiber: 1.4g
- ✓ Vitamin C: 4mg
- ✓ Antioxidants: Resveratrol

Apples:

Nutritional Information (per medium apple):

- ✓ Calories: 95
- ✓ Fiber: 4g
- ✓ Vitamin C: 14mg
- ✓ Antioxidants: Quercetin

Cherries:

Nutritional Information (per 1 cup, pitted):

- ✓ Calories: 87
- ✓ Fiber: 3g
- ✓ Vitamin C: 10mg
- ✓ Antioxidants: Anthocyanins

Bananas:

Nutritional Information (per medium banana):

- ✓ Calories: 105
- ✓ Fiber: 3.1g
- ✓ Vitamin C: 10mg
- ✓ Antioxidants: Dopamine

Pomegranates:

Nutritional Information (per 1 cup, arils):

- ✓ Calories: 83
- ✓ Fiber: 4g
- ✓ Vitamin C: 10mg
- ✓ Antioxidants: Punicalagins

CHAPTER 3

VEGETABLES

Spinach:

Nutritional Information (per 1 cup, raw):

- ✓ Calories: 7
- ✓ Fiber: 0.7g
- ✓ Vitamin K: 144mcg
- ✓ Folate: 58mcg

Kale:

Nutritional Information (per 1 cup, raw):

- ✓ Calories: 33
- ✓ Fiber: 2.4g
- ✓ Vitamin K: 547mcg
- ✓ Vitamin A: 547mcg

Broccoli:

Nutritional Information (per 1 cup, raw):

- ✓ Calories: 31
- ✓ Fiber: 2.4g
- ✓ Vitamin C: 81mg
- ✓ Folate: 53mcg

Carrots:

Nutritional Information (per 1 cup, raw):

- ✓ Calories: 52
- ✓ Fiber: 3.6g
- ✓ Vitamin A: 509mcg
- ✓ Vitamin K: 16mcg

Bell Peppers (Red):

Nutritional Information (per 1 cup, raw):

- ✓ Calories: 46
- ✓ Fiber: 3.6g
- ✓ Vitamin C: 190mg
- ✓ Vitamin A: 3726IU

Tomatoes:

Nutritional Information (per 1 cup, cherry tomatoes):

- ✓ Calories: 27
- ✓ Fiber: 2.2g
- ✓ Vitamin C: 24mg
- ✓ Lycopene: 3023mcg

Cauliflower:

Nutritional Information (per 1 cup, raw):

- ✓ Calories: 27
- ✓ Fiber: 2.5g
- ✓ Vitamin C: 51mg
- ✓ Folate: 55mcg

Brussels Sprouts:

Nutritional Information (per 1 cup, raw):

- ✓ Calories: 38
- ✓ Fiber: 3.3g
- ✓ Vitamin K: 156mcg
- ✓ Vitamin C: 75mg

Sweet Potatoes:

Nutritional Information (per 1 medium sweet potato):

- ✓ Calories: 103
- ✓ Fiber: 4g
- ✓ Vitamin A: 43896IU
- ✓ Vitamin C: 3.1mg

Avocado:

Nutritional Information (per 1 cup, sliced):

- ✓ Calories: 234
- ✓ Fiber: 12g
- ✓ Vitamin K: 42mcg
- ✓ Monounsaturated Fats: 20.9g

CHAPTER 4

WHOLE GRAINS

Quinoa:

Nutritional Information (per 1 cup, cooked):

- ✓ Calories: 222
- ✓ Fiber: 5.2g
- ✓ Protein: 8.1g
- ✓ Magnesium: 118mg

Oats:

Nutritional Information (per 1 cup, cooked):

- ✓ Calories: 147
- ✓ Fiber: 4g
- ✓ Protein: 6g
- ✓ Iron: 2.5mg

Brown Rice:

Nutritional Information (per 1 cup, cooked):

- ✓ Calories: 215
- ✓ Fiber: 3.5g
- ✓ Protein: 5g
- ✓ Magnesium: 86mg

Barley:

Nutritional Information (per 1 cup, cooked):

- ✓ Calories: 193
- ✓ Fiber: 6g
- ✓ Protein: 3.5g
- ✓ Magnesium: 79mg

Farro:

Nutritional Information (per 1 cup, cooked):

- ✓ Calories: 220
- ✓ Fiber: 7.9g
- ✓ Protein: 7.7g
- ✓ Magnesium: 68mg

Buckwheat:

Nutritional Information (per 1 cup, cooked):

- ✓ Calories: 154
- ✓ Fiber: 4.5g
- ✓ Protein: 6g
- ✓ Magnesium: 86mg

Quinoa:

Nutritional Information (per 1 cup, cooked):

- ✓ Calories: 222
- ✓ Fiber: 5.2g
- ✓ Protein: 8.1g
- ✓ Magnesium: 118mg

Whole Wheat Pasta:

Nutritional Information (per 1 cup, cooked):

- ✓ Calories: 174
- ✓ Fiber: 6.3g
- ✓ Protein: 7.5g
- ✓ Iron: 1.7mg

Millet:

Nutritional Information (per 1 cup, cooked):

- ✓ Calories: 207
- ✓ Fiber: 2.3g
- ✓ Protein: 6.1g
- ✓ Magnesium: 76mg

Amaranth:

Nutritional Information (per 1 cup, cooked):

- ✓ Calories: 251
- ✓ Fiber: 9.3g
- ✓ Protein: 9.3g
- ✓ Magnesium: 159mg

CHAPTER 5

FISH

Salmon:

Nutritional Information (per 3 ounces, cooked):

- ✓ Calories: 206
- ✓ Protein: 22g
- ✓ Omega-3 Fatty Acids: 1,226mg
- ✓ Vitamin D: 570IU

Mackerel:

Nutritional Information (per 3 ounces, cooked):

- ✓ Calories: 431
- ✓ Protein: 21g
- ✓ Omega-3 Fatty Acids: 4,580mg
- ✓ Vitamin D: 219IU

Sardines:

Nutritional Information (per 3 ounces, canned in oil, drained):

- ✓ Calories: 177
- ✓ Protein: 21g
- ✓ Omega-3 Fatty Acids: 1,480mg
- ✓ Vitamin D: 177IU

Trout:

Nutritional Information (per 3 ounces, cooked):

- ✓ Calories: 144
- ✓ Protein: 21g
- ✓ Omega-3 Fatty Acids: 1,040mg
- ✓ Vitamin D: 570IU

Herring:

Nutritional Information (per 3 ounces, cooked):

- ✓ Calories: 211
- ✓ Protein: 19g
- ✓ Omega-3 Fatty Acids: 1,722mg
- ✓ Vitamin D: 1,628IU

Tuna (Albacore):

Nutritional Information (per 3 ounces, canned in water):

- ✓ Calories: 109
- ✓ Protein: 20g
- ✓ Omega-3 Fatty Acids: 958mg
- ✓ Vitamin D: 150IU

Halibut:

Nutritional Information (per 3 ounces, cooked):

- ✓ Calories: 94
- ✓ Protein: 20g
- ✓ Omega-3 Fatty Acids: 490mg
- ✓ Vitamin D: 196IU

Cod:

Nutritional Information (per 3 ounces, cooked):

- ✓ Calories: 89
- ✓ Protein: 20g
- ✓ Omega-3 Fatty Acids: 83mg
- ✓ Vitamin D: 56IU

Shrimp:

Nutritional Information (per 3 ounces, cooked):

- ✓ Calories: 84
- ✓ Protein: 18g
- ✓ Omega-3 Fatty Acids: 259mg
- ✓ Vitamin D: 159IU

Anchovies:

Nutritional Information (per 2 ounces, canned in oil, drained):

Calories: 94

Protein: 14g

Omega-3 Fatty Acids: 1,000mg

Vitamin D: 253IU

CHAPTER 6

POULTRY

Chicken (Breast, Skinless):

Nutritional Information (per 3 ounces, cooked):

- ✓ Calories: 165
- ✓ Protein: 31g
- ✓ Total Fat: 3.6g
- ✓ Iron: 1mg

Turkey (Breast, Skinless):

Nutritional Information (per 3 ounces, cooked):

- ✓ Calories: 135
- ✓ Protein: 30g
- ✓ Total Fat: 1g
- ✓ Iron: 1.4mg

Duck (Breast, Skinless):

Nutritional Information (per 3 ounces, cooked):

- ✓ Calories: 135
- ✓ Protein: 23g
- ✓ Total Fat: 4g
- ✓ Iron: 2.3mg

Quail:

Nutritional Information (per 3 ounces, cooked):

- ✓ Calories: 134
- ✓ Protein: 22g
- ✓ Total Fat: 4g
- ✓ Iron: 2mg

Chicken (Thigh, Skinless):

Nutritional Information (per 3 ounces, cooked):

- ✓ Calories: 180
- ✓ Protein: 21g
- ✓ Total Fat: 9.3g
- ✓ Iron: 1.3mg

Turkey (Ground):

Nutritional Information (per 3 ounces, cooked):

- ✓ Calories: 193
- ✓ Protein: 20g
- ✓ Total Fat: 11g
- ✓ Iron: 1.8mg

Chicken (Leg, Skinless):

Nutritional Information (per 3 ounces, cooked):

- ✓ Calories: 174
- ✓ Protein: 28g
- ✓ Total Fat: 6.7g
- ✓ Iron: 2mg

Cornish Hen:

Nutritional Information (per 3 ounces, cooked):

- ✓ Calories: 136
- ✓ Protein: 25g
- ✓ Total Fat: 4.5g
- ✓ Iron: 1.5mg

Turkey (Thigh, Skinless):

Nutritional Information (per 3 ounces, cooked):

- ✓ Calories: 180
- ✓ Protein: 22g
- ✓ Total Fat: 10g
- ✓ Iron: 1.6mg

Chicken (Ground):

Nutritional Information (per 3 ounces, cooked):

- ✓ Calories: 187
- ✓ Protein: 20g
- ✓ Total Fat: 11g
- ✓ Iron: 1.8mg

CHAPTER 7

OLIVE OIL

Extra Virgin Olive Oil:

Nutritional Information (per 1 tablespoon):

- ✓ Calories: 120
- ✓ Total Fat: 14g
- ✓ Saturated Fat: 2g
- ✓ Monounsaturated Fat: 10g
- ✓ Polyunsaturated Fat: 1.5g
- ✓ Vitamin E: 1.9mg

Virgin Olive Oil:

Nutritional Information (per 1 tablespoon):

- ✓ Calories: 119
- ✓ Total Fat: 14g
- ✓ Saturated Fat: 2g
- ✓ Monounsaturated Fat: 10g
- ✓ Polyunsaturated Fat: 1.5g
- ✓ Vitamin E: 1.9mg

Pure Olive Oil:

Nutritional Information (per 1 tablespoon):

- ✓ Calories: 119
- ✓ Total Fat: 13.5g
- ✓ Saturated Fat: 2g
- ✓ Monounsaturated Fat: 9.8g
- ✓ Polyunsaturated Fat: 1.4g
- ✓ Vitamin E: 1.9mg

Light Olive Oil:

Nutritional Information (per 1 tablespoon):

- ✓ Calories: 120
- ✓ Total Fat: 14g
- ✓ Saturated Fat: 2g
- ✓ Monounsaturated Fat: 10g
- ✓ Polyunsaturated Fat: 1.5g
- ✓ Vitamin E: 1.9mg

Organic Extra Virgin Olive Oil:

Nutritional Information (per 1 tablespoon):

- ✓ Calories: 119
- ✓ Total Fat: 14g
- ✓ Saturated Fat: 2g
- ✓ Monounsaturated Fat: 10g
- ✓ Polyunsaturated Fat: 1.5g
- ✓ Vitamin E: 1.9mg

Cold-Pressed Olive Oil:

Nutritional Information (per 1 tablespoon):

- ✓ Calories: 119
- ✓ Total Fat: 13.5g
- ✓ Saturated Fat: 2g
- ✓ Monounsaturated Fat: 9.8g
- ✓ Polyunsaturated Fat: 1.4g
- ✓ Vitamin E: 1.9mg

Spanish Olive Oil:

Nutritional Information (per 1 tablespoon):

- ✓ Calories: 119
- ✓ Total Fat: 14g
- ✓ Saturated Fat: 2g
- ✓ Monounsaturated Fat: 10g
- ✓ Polyunsaturated Fat: 1.5g
- ✓ Vitamin E: 1.9mg

Italian Olive Oil:

Nutritional Information (per 1 tablespoon):

- ✓ Calories: 119
- ✓ Total Fat: 14g
- ✓ Saturated Fat: 2g
- ✓ Monounsaturated Fat: 10g
- ✓ Polyunsaturated Fat: 1.5g
- ✓ Vitamin E: 1.9mg

Greek Olive Oil:

Nutritional Information (per 1 tablespoon):

- ✓ Calories: 119
- ✓ Total Fat: 14g
- ✓ Saturated Fat: 2g
- ✓ Monounsaturated Fat: 10g
- ✓ Polyunsaturated Fat: 1.5g
- ✓ Vitamin E: 1.9mg

Infused Olive Oil (e.g., garlic-infused):

Nutritional Information (per 1 tablespoon):

- ✓ Calories: 120
- ✓ Total Fat: 14g
- ✓ Saturated Fat: 2g
- ✓ Monounsaturated Fat: 10g
- ✓ Polyunsaturated Fat: 1.5g
- ✓ Vitamin E: 1.9mg

CHAPTER 8

FOODS TO LIMIT OR AVOID

Red Meat (Beef):

Nutritional Information (per 3 ounces, cooked):

- ✓ Calories: 213
- ✓ Total Fat: 11g
- ✓ Saturated Fat: 4g
- ✓ Protein: 29g

Processed Meats (Hot Dogs, Sausages):

Nutritional Information (per 1 hot dog):

- ✓ Calories: 150
- ✓ Total Fat: 13g
- ✓ Saturated Fat: 5g
- ✓ Protein: 5g

Butter:

Nutritional Information (per 1 tablespoon):

- ✓ Calories: 102
- ✓ Total Fat: 12g
- ✓ Saturated Fat: 7g
- ✓ Cholesterol: 31mg

Cheese (Full-Fat):

Nutritional Information (per 1 ounce):

- ✓ Calories: 110
- ✓ Total Fat: 9g
- ✓ Saturated Fat: 6g
- ✓ Protein: 7g

Fried Foods:

Nutritional Information (varies):

- ✓ Calories: Varies
- ✓ Total Fat: Varies
- ✓ Saturated Fat: Varies
- ✓ Trans Fat: Varies

Fast Food (Burgers, Fries):

Nutritional Information (varies):

- ✓ Calories: Varies
- ✓ Total Fat: Varies
- ✓ Saturated Fat: Varies
- ✓ Trans Fat: Varies

Pastries (Cakes, Cookies):

Nutritional Information (varies):

- ✓ Calories: Varies
- ✓ Total Fat: Varies
- ✓ Saturated Fat: Varies
- ✓ Sugar: Varies

Sweets (Candy, Sugary Snacks):

Nutritional Information (varies):

- ✓ Calories: Varies
- ✓ Total Fat: Varies
- ✓ Saturated Fat: Varies
- ✓ Sugar: Varies

Ice Cream:

Nutritional Information (per 1/2 cup):

- ✓ Calories: 137
- ✓ Total Fat: 7g
- ✓ Saturated Fat: 4g
- ✓ Sugar: 14g

Potato Chips:

Nutritional Information (per 1 ounce):

- ✓ Calories: 152
- ✓ Total Fat: 10g
- ✓ Saturated Fat: 3g
- ✓ Sodium: 95mg

Soda (Regular):

Nutritional Information (per 12 ounces):

- ✓ Calories: 140
- ✓ Total Sugars: 39g
- ✓ Sodium: 30mg

White Bread:

Nutritional Information (per slice):

- ✓ Calories: 70
- ✓ Total Carbohydrates: 14g
- ✓ Dietary Fiber: 1g
- ✓ Protein: 2g

White Rice:

Nutritional Information (per 1 cup, cooked):

- ✓ Calories: 204
- ✓ Total Carbohydrates: 45g
- ✓ Protein: 4g
- ✓ Fiber: 1g

Highly Processed Snacks (Chips, Crackers):

Nutritional Information (varies):

- ✓ Calories: Varies
- ✓ Total Fat: Varies
- ✓ Saturated Fat: Varies
- ✓ Sodium: Varies

Margarine:

Nutritional Information (per 1 tablespoon):

- ✓ Calories: 102
- ✓ Total Fat: 12g
- ✓ Saturated Fat: 2g
- ✓ Trans Fat: 2g

Microwave Popcorn (Butter-flavored):

Nutritional Information (per 3 cups, popped):

- ✓ Calories: 93
- ✓ Total Fat: 7g
- ✓ Saturated Fat: 1g
- ✓ Sodium: 146mg

Canned Soup (High Sodium):

Nutritional Information (varies):

- ✓ Calories: Varies
- ✓ Total Fat: Varies
- ✓ Saturated Fat: Varies
- ✓ Sodium: Varies

Energy Drinks:

Nutritional Information (per 8 ounces):

- ✓ Calories: 110
- ✓ Total Sugars: 27g
- ✓ Caffeine: Varies

Alcohol (Excessive):

Nutritional Information (varies):

- ✓ Calories: Varies
- ✓ Alcohol Content: Varies

Highly Processed Lunch Meats:

Nutritional Information (per 2 slices):

- ✓ Calories: Varies
- ✓ Total Fat: Varies
- ✓ Saturated Fat: Varies
- ✓ Sodium: Varies

CONCLUSION

As we draw the curtain on this odyssey through the aromatic realms of the MIND diet, let the echoes of rejuvenated minds linger in the spaces between these pages. The alchemy of carefully curated ingredients, the symphony of flavors resonating with the promise of cognitive vitality – it is a tale that transcends the ordinary and touches the very fabric of our existence.

In the gentle embrace of berries, the crisp crunch of leafy greens, and the delicate dance of nuts and fish, we find not just sustenance but a communion with the essence of well-being. The MIND diet is more than a mere culinary guide; it is a testament to the resilience of the human spirit, a celebration of the harmony between nutrition and cognitive health.

As you embark on your own culinary journey through the pages of this book, remember that each recipe is a brushstroke in the portrait of your well-being. Let the kitchen become a sanctuary, and let each dish be an offering to the temple of your mind. For in the tapestry of flavors, we discover not just the richness of taste but the richness of life.

But this journey is not confined to these pages alone; it extends into the kitchens and lives of those who embrace it. Your feedback, your stories, and your experiences are the threads that weave this narrative into a living tapestry. I invite you to share your journey, your triumphs, and even your challenges. Let this be a dialogue, a shared exploration into the boundless potential of mindful nutrition.

Have you experienced the transformative power of the MIND diet? How has it touched your life, and what symphony of flavors resonates with the chords of your well-being? Your insights are not just valuable; they are the heartbeat of this ongoing conversation. Like a river flowing through the canyons of collective experience, your feedback nourishes the landscape of knowledge and understanding.

In closing, let the MIND diet not be a mere collection of recipes but a companion in your quest for a healthier, more vibrant life. As the aroma of the dishes lingers in your kitchen, may it also permeate the spaces of your mind, awakening the senses to the possibilities that lie within each carefully chosen ingredient.

Thank you for embarking on this journey with me. May your culinary endeavors be filled with joy, your minds be adorned with clarity, and your well-being be a testament to the poetry of mindful living. I eagerly await the notes of your experiences, the melodies of your discoveries, and the harmonies of your feedback. Together, let us continue to compose the symphony of a life well-nourished.

BONUS:

10 MIND DIET RECIPES

Berry Spinach Salad

Cooking Time: 15 minutes

Serving: 4

Ingredients:

- ✓ 6 cups fresh spinach leaves
- ✓ 1 cup strawberries, sliced.
- ✓ 1 cup blueberries
- ✓ 1/2 cup walnuts, chopped.
- ✓ 1/4 cup feta cheese, crumbled.
- ✓ Balsamic vinaigrette dressing

Instructions:

1. In a large bowl, combine spinach, strawberries, blueberries, walnuts, and feta cheese.
2. Drizzle with balsamic vinaigrette and toss gently.
3. Serve immediately.

Nutritional Information:

calories, 12g carbs, 4g protein, 10g fat, 4g fiber

Baked Salmon with Lemon and Dill

Cooking Time: 20 minutes

Serving: 2

Ingredients:

- ✓ 2 salmon fillets
- ✓ 1 lemon, sliced.
- ✓ 2 tablespoons fresh dill, chopped.
- ✓ Salt and pepper to taste
- ✓ Olive oil

Instructions:

1. Preheat oven to 400°F (200°C).
2. Place salmon fillets on a baking sheet.
3. Season with salt, pepper, and chopped dill. Top with lemon slices.
4. Drizzle with olive oil and bake for 15-18 minutes or until salmon is cooked through.

Nutritional Information:

300 calories, 0g carbs, 40g protein, 15g fat, 0g fiber

Quinoa and Vegetable Stir-Fry

Cooking Time: 25 minutes

Serving: 4

Ingredients:

- ✓ 1 cup quinoa, cooked.
- ✓ 2 cups broccoli florets
- ✓ 1 bell pepper, sliced.
- ✓ 1 carrot, julienned
- ✓ 1 cup snap peas
- ✓ 2 tablespoons soy sauce
- ✓ 1 tablespoon sesame oil

Instructions:

1. In a wok or large pan, sauté broccoli, bell pepper, carrot, and snap peas until crisp-tender.
2. Add cooked quinoa and stir in soy sauce and sesame oil.
3. Cook for an additional 3-5 minutes, stirring frequently.

Nutritional Information:

250 calories, 45g carbs, 10g protein, 5g fat, 6g fiber

Greek Yogurt Parfait

Preparation Time: 10 minutes

Serving: 1

Ingredients:

- ✓ 1 cup Greek yogurt
- ✓ 1/2 cup mixed berries (blueberries, strawberries)
- ✓ 2 tablespoons honey
- ✓ 1/4 cup granola

Instructions:

1. In a glass or bowl, layer Greek yogurt, mixed berries, and granola.
2. Drizzle with honey.
3. Repeat layers as desired.

Nutritional Information:

300 calories, 40g carbs, 20g protein, 8g fat, 5g fiber

Lentil and Vegetable Soup

Cooking Time: 30 minutes

Serving: 6

Ingredients:

- ✓ 1 cup dried green lentils
- ✓ 1 onion, diced.
- ✓ 2 carrots, sliced.
- ✓ 2 celery stalks, chopped.
- ✓ 3 cloves garlic, minced.
- ✓ 1 can (14 oz) diced tomatoes.
- ✓ 6 cups vegetable broth
- ✓ 1 teaspoon cumin
- ✓ Salt and pepper to taste

Instructions:

1. Rinse lentils and combine with vegetables, garlic, tomatoes, and broth in a large pot.
2. Add cumin, salt, and pepper. Bring to a boil, then simmer for 20-25 minutes.
3. Adjust seasonings as needed before serving.

Nutritional Information:

220 calories, 40g carbs, 15g protein, 1g fat, 15g fiber

Grilled Chicken and Vegetable Skewers

Cooking Time: 20 minutes

Serving: 4

Ingredients:

- ✓ 1 lb chicken breast, cubed.
- ✓ 2 zucchinis, sliced.
- ✓ 1 red onion, cut into chunks.
- ✓ Cherry tomatoes
- ✓ Olive oil
- ✓ Italian seasoning
- ✓ Salt and pepper to taste

Instructions:

1. Thread chicken, zucchini, onion, and tomatoes onto skewers.
2. Brush with olive oil and sprinkle with Italian seasoning, salt, and pepper.
3. Grill for 10-12 minutes, turning occasionally, until chicken is cooked through.

Nutritional Information:

280 calories, 10g carbs, 30g protein, 14g fat, 3g fiber

Spinach and Feta Stuffed Mushrooms

Cooking Time: 25 minutes

Serving: 8

Ingredients:

- ✓ 16 large mushrooms cleaned, and stems removed.
- ✓ 2 cups fresh spinach, chopped.
- ✓ 1/2 cup feta cheese, crumbled.
- ✓ 2 cloves garlic, minced.
- ✓ 1 tablespoon olive oil
- ✓ Salt and pepper to taste

Instructions:

1. Preheat oven to 375°F (190°C).
2. In a pan, sauté spinach and garlic in olive oil until wilted.
3. Mix in feta cheese and season with salt and pepper.
4. Stuff mushrooms with the spinach and feta mixture.
5. Bake for 15 minutes or until mushrooms are tender.

Nutritional Information:

90 calories, 5g carbs, 6g protein, 7g fat, 2g fiber

Mediterranean Chickpea Salad

Preparation Time: 15 minutes

Serving: 4

Ingredients:

- ✓ 2 cans (15 oz each) chickpeas, drained and rinsed.
- ✓ 1 cucumber, diced.
- ✓ 1 cup cherry tomatoes, halved.
- ✓ 1/2 red onion finely chopped.
- ✓ 1/4 cup Kalamata olives, sliced.
- ✓ 1/4 cup feta cheese, crumbled.
- ✓ Olive oil and lemon juice dressing
- ✓ Fresh parsley, chopped.

Instructions:

1. In a large bowl, combine chickpeas, cucumber, tomatoes, red onion, olives, and feta cheese.
2. Drizzle with olive oil and lemon juice dressing.
3. Garnish with fresh parsley before serving.

Nutritional Information:

320 calories, 45g carbs, 15g protein, 10g fat, 10g fiber

Sweet Potato and Chickpea Curry

Cooking Time: 30 minutes

Serving: 4

Ingredients:

- ✓ 2 sweet potatoes peeled and diced.
- ✓ 1 can (15 oz) chickpeas, drained and rinsed.
- ✓ 1 onion, chopped.
- ✓ 3 cloves garlic, minced.
- ✓ 1 can (14 oz) diced tomatoes.
- ✓ 1 can (14 oz) coconut milk
- ✓ 2 tablespoons curry powder
- ✓ Salt and pepper to taste

Instructions:

1. In a pot, sauté onion and garlic until softened.
2. Add sweet potatoes, chickpeas, diced tomatoes, coconut milk, and curry powder.
3. Season with salt and pepper. Simmer until sweet potatoes are tender.

Nutritional Information:

280 calories, 40g carbs, 8g protein, 12g fat, 8g fiber

Almond-Crusted Tilapia

Cooking Time: 15 minutes

Serving: 2

Ingredients:

- ✓ 2 tilapia fillets
- ✓ 1/2 cup almonds finely chopped.
- ✓ 1/4 cup whole wheat breadcrumbs
- ✓ 1 teaspoon lemon zest
- ✓ 1/2 teaspoon dried thyme
- ✓ Salt and pepper to taste
- ✓ Olive oil for baking

Instructions:

1. Preheat oven to 400°F (200°C).
2. In a bowl, mix chopped almonds, breadcrumbs, lemon zest, thyme, salt, and pepper.
3. Dip tilapia fillets in the almond mixture, pressing gently to adhere.
4. Place on a baking sheet, drizzle with olive oil, and bake for 12-15 minutes.

Nutritional Information:

280 calories, 10g carbs, 30g protein, 15g fat, 4g fiber

www.ingramcontent.com/pod-product-compliance
Lightning Source LLC
Chambersburg PA
CBHW070118010626
45794CB00013B/2575